When the Doctor Says IT'S CANCER

MARY BETH MOSTER

POCKET GUIDES
Tyndale House Publishers, Inc.
Wheaton, Illinois

Adapted from *Living with Cancer*, © 1979 by Mary Beth Moster, published by Tyndale House Publishers, Inc.

Scripture references are taken from the *New American Standard Bible*, © 1960, 1962, 1963, 1968, 1971, 1973, and 1975 by The Lockman Foundation, unless otherwise indicated.

First printing, October 1986
Library of Congress Catalog Card Number 86-50656
ISBN 0-8423-7981-9
© 1986 by Mary Beth Moster

CONTENTS

Introduction:
The Diagnosis We Dread   5

ONE
What Is Cancer?   9

TWO
Cures and Their Side Effects   15

THREE
How Cancer Affects Your Self-Image   21

FOUR
Facing Negative Emotions 30

FIVE
The Hopeful Side of Death 43

SIX
Ten Questions Families Ask   54

SEVEN
Children with Cancer 66

Fifteen Common Sites of Cancer 77

Helping Agencies   91

Notes   92

The Diagnosis We Dread

It was a beautiful wedding. The candles flickered, casting a warm glow through the pews filled with friends and loved ones. At the sound of the wedding march, all eyes turned to Jan. Her dark eyes were shining and happy, and Greg's heart beat faster as she neared. She carried roses and daisies.

Neither of them knew then that Jan's life would be like the spring flowers in her hands—lovely, full of life, but gone far too soon.

Greg is my husband's brother. All of us in the family loved Jan from the time he first brought her home for us to meet. We were happy for them as we saw their love deepen and grow stronger. They dreamed of a house and children and a lifetime together.

Not quite two years after the wedding, Jan became ill. Nausea, double vision, numbness in one arm. Was it flu? The headaches were unbearable. Was it nerves? Doctors were consulted, but they had trouble diagnosing the problem. Soon it became clear that something was seriously wrong. At last, surgery. Then an answer.

Diagnosis: brain tumor, malignant.

This lovely girl was not yet twenty-five. All her hopes for her future came crashing down around her. Her dreams of being the mother of a houseful of children were gone. As health ebbed from her, so did her physical beauty.

As the rest of us stumbled through those long, agonizing months, we saw the stark reality of human tragedy. We witnessed the anguish of her mother and father, the heartbreak Greg was suffering. We grieved with Jan as the days passed and the hope for recovery slipped away.

THE MOST FEARED DISEASE

Cancer is often called the most feared disease and I believe the description is true. A thousand people die from cancer every day in our land.

Jan was the victim of one of the most dreaded and devastating forms of cancer. Her neurosurgeon told us the type of malignancy she had was extremely fast-growing and not one that ordinarily responds well to treatment. She lived about a year and a half after diagnosis.

What Jan experienced is an example of what we all fear; but today, as never before, there is hope of cure for many forms of cancer. Millions of people who have encountered the disease live many normal, active years after proper treatment. A large number of those people are eventually pronounced cured.

But regardless of its long-term effects, cancer wreaks havoc in the lives of its victims, family members, and friends. Every time I read the statistics about the millions of people with cancer in this country, I know that each number represents a home gripped by the icy fingers of fear.

I began to see a need for a book for cancer patients, their families, and others concerned about the lives touched by this particular disease. The aim of *When the Doctor Says, "It's Cancer"* is to:

- explain some of the medical aspects of cancer
- face examples of the practical problems often encountered
- look at common emotional responses experienced by cancer patients and their families
- show the tremendous resource a faith in God can be during crisis.

It is my hope that this book will help cancer patients in any situation.

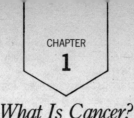

What Is Cancer?

Cancer is no respecter of persons. It strikes young, old, rich, poor, all races and religions, beauty queens and wallflowers. People in all parts of the world have it in some form.

The United Cancer Council tells us that cancer is not even limited to people. Dogs and cats can get it. Wild animals, reptiles, plants, and insects all can get cancer.

Cancer Fact
- 930,000 Americans are diagnosed as having cancer each year.

The American Cancer Society (ACS) reports that about 73 million Americans now living will eventually have cancer; that is about 30 percent, according to present rates. Over the years, cancer will strike in approximately three out of four families.

Nearly everyone, it seems, will encounter cancer someday, either personally or in the life of a loved one.

But today we have real hope for cure.

"There are over five million Americans alive today," says the ACS, "who have a history of cancer, three million of them with a diagnosis five or more years ago." Most of these three million can be considered cured. One out of three people treated for cancer now has a normal life expectancy; it should soon be one out of two, due in large part to early detection.

Great advances have been made in the treatment of certain types of cancer. Hodgkin's disease, Wilms' tumor, acute lymphocytic leukemia, and testicular cancer are among those cancers that are treated with more promising results than ever before.

WHAT IS IT, ANYWAY?

The word *cancer* is used to describe an uncontrolled growth of abnormal cells. The United Cancer Council says:

> A body is made up of billions of normal cells, all of which multiply and divide in an orderly manner to perform their own particular functions. Whenever these cells, for some as yet unknown reason, go berserk and grow in a disorderly and chaotic manner, crowding out normal cells and robbing them of nourishment, the condition is known as cancer.[1]

The disease creeps into a life insidiously, normally without pain until it is advanced.

Some cancers are more serious than others. Some are fast growing, spreading in several weeks. Others grow slowly, multiplying over several years. Cancer can start in any tissue of the body.

Some cancers are discovered early, before they have spread. Others are located in places in the body where certain treatments—surgery and radiation therapy, for example—are difficult, if not impossible. In many sites, however, cancer is curable by these techniques if detected early.

The ACS states flatly, "Cancer is a group of diseases in which there is uncontrolled growth of abnormal cells, which, if unchecked, will cause death."[2] Because of this fact, it is important that surgery and other recommended treatments are not delayed.

Though researchers have been trying to find the causes of the disease, the task is

The Tenacious Disease

Hippocrates first identified cancer about 400 B.C. He divided tumors into two large groups, the "innocuous" (or benign) and "dangerous" (or malignant). He also coined the term *karkinoma* (meaning "crab") for solid, malignant tumors. The Latin word for "crab," *cancrum*, was later the basis for our word *cancer*. No one is sure why Hippocrates chose the word *crab* to describe malignant tumors, but some people guess it is because the crab grabs hold of its prey with such tenacity.

difficult because cancer behaves in so many different ways. Some cancers have been induced in animals; this has led scientists to believe that in the future it might be possible to vaccinate against a few forms of the disease. More and more scientists are becoming convinced that in many cases cancer is environmentally induced.

TERMS YOU NEED TO KNOW

Each type of cancer is normally defined by the place, or site, in the body where it is growing. The appendix in this book contains detailed information on the most frequent sites of the disease in humans.

Cancer is further defined by the biological characteristics of the tumor. Not all tumors are malignant. A *benign* tumor, though abnormal, is rarely dangerous to a person's life. It grows to a certain size and then stops growing; it does not spread.

A *malignant* (cancerous) tumor, on the other hand, keeps on growing. The cells from the original site of the cancer can dislodge, be carried by the bloodstream or lymphatic systems to other parts of the body and give rise to additional tumors. *Metastasis* is the process of the spread of cancer. Without treatment cancerous cells will eventually invade vital organs, robbing them of nourishment.

Two words are frequently used in cancer diagnosis: *carcinoma* and *sarcoma*. Carcinomas are cancers of epithelial tissues.

These are tissues that cover a surface, line a cavity, or protect a surface. The external surfaces of the body (skin, breast) and internal surfaces (alimentary tract, organs such as the liver, pancreas, intestines, prostate, thyroid) are all subject to carcinomas. Sarcomas are cancers arising in any connective tissue (muscles, cartilage, bone, etc.).

A physician suspicious of cancer will order a number of tests, but the most accurate test used is the *biopsy*. In this test a sample of tissue is removed and examined chemically and microscopically.

Usually, when a person dies from cancer, the malignant tumor itself is not the direct cause of death. Bowel obstruction, kidney failure, perforation, bleeding and infections are some of the complications of malignancies that can bring about the death of the patient.

When cancer is diagnosed, the patient might come under the care of a hematologist/oncologist: *Hematology* is the study of the blood; *oncology* is the study of tumors.

Sometimes following treatment of cancer a patient experiences a *remission*, a state wherein the symptoms of the disease are not manifested. Being in remission is not the same as being cured, because the cancer cells are still in the body, even if they cannot be seen through a microscope.

Check Your Cancer IQ

Indicate whether you think the following statements are true or false. Statements refer to cancer in the United States.

1. There is no scientific proof that cancer in humans is contagious.
2. Cancer is the second most frequent cause of death in the United States.
3. In the treatment of cancer, it is usually better to use one method of treatment rather than a combination of methods.
4. Cancers sometime grow so rapidly that treatment, such as surgery or chemotherapy, should be started as soon as possible.
5. One out of every three people who get cancer is currently being saved.
6. While there is no evidence that cancer is inherited, there is some evidence that susceptibility to cancer may be inherited.
7. One out of every three persons living in the United States today at some time in his/her life will develop cancer.
8. The most common cancer in women is cancer of the breast.
9. The most common cancer in men is cancer of the lung.
10. All cancer is caused by a nutritional deficiency.
11. Cancer is not always curable but it is often treatable.
12. Cancer is largely a preventable disease.

Answers: 1.T, 2.T, 3.F, 4.T, 5.T, 6.T, 7.T, 8.F, 9.T, 10.F, 11.T, 12.T.

(From *Understanding Cancer* by Steven Leib and Merk Rennecker. Reprinted by permission of Bull Publishing Co., P. O. Box 208, Palo Alto, CA 94302.)

CHAPTER 2

Cures and
Their Side Effects

Until this century there was little hope for the cancer patient; death was inevitable. But today the outlook is much brighter. With early diagnosis and proper treatment, more and more people are saved from cancer every year. Using chemotherapy, surgery, and radiation therapy, either as a single treatment or in sophisticated combinations with other measures, cancer is now considered one of the *most curable diseases in this country.*

Surgery is one of the most significant treatments for the disease, and it is always recommended wherever possible.

Radiation therapy effectively <u>stops the growth</u> of cancer cells in certain types of cancers. About half of all cancer patients are treated with radiation, either alone or in combination with other therapy.

Beyond these two measures, cancer is now being successfully treated by radioactive substances, various drugs, chemicals, and hormones. The treatment of cancer is extremely complex, but basically the intent is to remove cancer cells by surgery or to destroy them (or inhibit reproduction) with radiation or chemotherapy.

SURGERY

Cancer does not always mean a change in lifestyle. A cancer patient often is able to return to work and other daily activities without the treatment for cancer greatly affecting his day-to-day routine.

But sometimes this is not the case. Radical surgery can cause serious problems of adjustment:

- Patients with colon-rectum cancer may need to adjust to wearing a colostomy bag.
- Breast cancer surgery usually involves the loss of the breast and surrounding tissue.
- Laryngectomees often need to learn to talk without vocal cords.
- Bone cancer patients sometimes must lose an arm or leg and then learn to use an artificial limb.

Most people who have surgery that changes the body image or a body function will go through a period of great distress and depression. If the cancer patient has lost a part of his body, he will mourn that loss. His grief will be much like what he would experience if a loved one had died. The loss is permanent.

One salesman said, "I knew I had to lose my vocal cords in order to live—I just wasn't sure I wanted to live without my vocal cords. After all, my business, my livelihood, depended on my ability to talk." After long and difficult months of training, he has now learned esophageal speech and is adjusting to his loss.

Many people have limitations of this kind thrust on them within a few days or hours of diagnosis. The result of the cancer is visible and drastic. It is even more of a shock because the symptoms had often seemed barely significant enough to call to the doctor's attention. One woman said, "I just couldn't believe that tiny lump could change things so drastically."

Surgery for cancer sometimes must be extensive and radical to remove all tissue to which the cancer may have spread. In *Science against Cancer*, Pat McGrady says that surgical techniques, enhanced by new anesthetics, more effective antibiotics to control infection, transfusions, and rigid sterile precautions are now permitting operative procedures that would have been impossible a few years ago.[1]

RADIATION THERAPY

In radiation, too, remarkable strides have been made. Such instruments as linear accelerators, betatrons, and radioactive cobalt-60 teletherapy apparatus have become standard equipment for treating deep-seated cancers.

Radiation therapy uses ionizing radiations

to destroy cells by injuring their capacity to divide. Some cancers are more responsive to radiation than others. The new radiation instruments produce energy in the multi-million electron volt range and can deliver a greater dose of radiation to deep-seated tumors without the discomfort and skin reactions that often accompany the lower-energy X-ray beams.

CHEMOTHERAPY

Twenty-five years ago, chemotherapy was reserved for the cancer patient with widespread metastases and little hope of recovery. It was a last-ditch effort.

Today, chemotherapy plays a major role in the early treatment of cancer. It is a standard form of therapy, and oncologists use it routinely with the goal of curing the patient.

Susan Golden in *Nursing Forum* gives the reason for the optimism: "Three major advances in cancer chemotherapy have contributed to this new perspective: (1) the development of new drugs, (2) the concept of combined-agent chemotherapy, and (3) the use of drug therapy in conjunction with radiation and surgery for early cancer patients with poor prognosis."

She notes that doctors have a choice of at least eighty anti-tumor drugs available, while new drugs are being developed steadily.[2]

The drugs used in chemotherapy act in two basic ways: either they kill tumor cells (cytocidal), or else they create conditions adverse to cell reproduction (cytostatic). These drugs are used with an exact knowledge of the cell cycle to get the maximum destruction of malignant cells at the varying stages of cell growth, while at the same time doing as little damage as possible to normal cells. Inevitably, though, normal cells will also be affected by the chemotherapy, and various side effects will result.

The drugs used in chemotherapy are designed to destroy the rapidly reproducing cancer cells. Therefore, the normal cells that naturally reproduce quickly will usually be the ones adversely affected by the drugs. The digestive tract, hair roots, and bone marrow all have actively reproducing cells; this is why it is common for patients on chemotherapy to lose their hair and have nausea, exhaustion, diarrhea, mouth and lip ulcers, and blood-related problems (anemia, insufficient white cell count, hemorrhage, etc.).

Not everyone has side effects, and sometimes these discomforts last just a few days. If the reaction to the drug is very severe, the physician may want to reduce the dosage or discontinue the drug altogether.

TWO SIDE EFFECTS

1. *Hair loss*. Hair loss can occur from both radiation and certain drugs used in chemotherapy. This is one of the most devastating side effects of treatment, and it is

especially difficult for teenagers and young adults. This side effect is not dangerous, but it can be emotionally upsetting. The patient should be prepared well in advance so that he or she will know what is probably going to happen.

It is good to talk about getting a wig early, and a trip should be made to the barbershop or beauty shop before the loss is complete. Wigs are so common now for both men and women that a selection can be made with relative ease. The payment for these wigs is covered by most insurance policies. Eyebrow pencils and false eyelashes can also be purchased. The hair does grow back again after therapy, but it takes several months.

2. *Weakness*. Many cancer patients experience unusual lack of energy after radiation or chemotherapy. To people who are normally vibrant, this weakness is especially frustrating.

One working mother says: "It's all I can do to get through the day at work—I'm just so worn out. Then I come home and look around and see all the dust, and the sweeper needs to be run, and I just feel like giving up. My husband and the girls are great about pitching in and helping, but it still frustrates me that I can't do it myself. I'd also like to have company over for dinner sometimes, but I never know if I'll feel up to it, so we just never invite anyone."

CHAPTER 3

How Cancer Affects Your Self-Image

What gives a person a sense of worth? Of value as a human being?

Psychologists have spent long years studying the phenomenon of self-esteem in an effort to determine the factors involved in a person's opinion of himself.

The factors are many and varied. They involve such attributes as physical appearance, intelligence, character, the ability to work and be productive, and the ability to compensate for real or imagined shortcomings.

What are the main stresses placed on a cancer patient's self-esteem? How can he cope with them?

A NEW BODY IMAGE

We cannot escape the emphasis our culture places on beauty—sheer, physical, skin-deep beauty. If we cannot be beautiful, our culture then insists that we at least not be "disfigured" or "abnormal" or "different" in any way. James Dobson, Ph.D., says, "Without question, the most highly valued personal attribute in our culture (and in most others) is physical attractiveness."[1]

This cultural emphasis on physical perfection is one of the first concerns of the cancer patient. He asks, "What will happen to my body?"

Breast cancer has been the object of a great amount of publicity recently, mainly because of the national attention given the wives of several political figures who talked openly about their mastectomies. Their frankness has been instrumental in partially removing the cloak of secrecy that has in the past surrounded breast cancer.

Rene C. Mastrovito, M.D., of the Memorial Sloan-Kettering Cancer Center in New York, explains how mastectomy surgery is more devastating for some women than others:

> The psychological assault of a radical mastectomy is greater on some women than it is on others. A woman whose concept of self-worth is significantly and strongly dependent upon her sense of femininity and her female body image will have suffered a greater loss than will a woman whose personal identification makes this attribute less important.[2]

A SOCIAL STIGMA
Eileen Tiedt, in *Nursing Forum*, says, "Our society places an enormous stigma on cancer. . . . Because of the stigma attached

to cancer and the value placed on the intact, healthy body, cancer patients do not readily talk about what has and is happening to them." She says sometimes a patient's emotional energy is spent helping others cope with their emotional response to his situation, rather than coping with his own needs.[3]

One exceptionally healthy-looking man in the prime of life chooses to tell no one other than his wife about his cancer. He knows of the stigma attached to the disease, and he wants no one to treat him differently or with pity. As Rene Mastrovito says:

> Cancer is a source of severe psychological as well as somatic [bodily] stress. It is a feared disease because it implies a fatal outcome. It is a dreaded disease because of projected fears of pain, body damage, deterioration and invalidism. It is a repugnant disease because it imbues the victim with a certain sense of being unclean and unwholesome. Finally it is a condition that may engender an overpowering sense of helplessness. . . .[4]

AN EMOTIONAL DRAIN

A person's self-esteem is vitally affected by his emotional responses to difficult or life-threatening circumstances. Maurice E. Wagner, Th.M., Ph.D., describes the stress a person might encounter when he is given a diagnosis of cancer:

> Our self-concept may seem fairly stable when life's ebb and flow of problems stays within

acceptable limits. Occasionally, however, a tidal wave of unexpected difficulties over-whelms us. It may be a surprise illness, the sudden death of a loved one, a business failure, or a marriage or family problem we cannot handle. Our boat is not only rocked: it seems as if it is about to split in the middle and take water.[5]

SHAKEN SELF-ESTEEM: HOW WE COPE

Just to get along in day-to-day life we all use what psychiatrists refer to as "coping mechanisms." These are, Mastrovito says, various "strategies, behavior patterns, at-titudes, and personal physical and emotional attributes which are used in dealing with one's self and the environment. Where suc-cessful, these life patterns maintain self-esteem, acceptability by others and a sense of mastery over one's destiny."[6]

You will notice that physical attributes are mentioned among the coping mechanisms that contribute to a sense of self-esteem. If a physical attribute is changed or removed due to the cancer, the patient has lost an important psychological coping mechanism. Of course, each person's situation is unique. A simple, isolated, and uncomplicated cancer might be removed completely and cause the patient no further distress. Other patients might experience the tremendous stress of catastrophe such as paralysis or blindness.

What coping mechanisms are available to the cancer patient who is experiencing blows to his self-esteem?

Denial. Probably every cancer patient, at one time or another, uses the coping mechanism of denial.

"Denial," says Mastrovito, "is not necessarily a pathological condition. Since it is a protective mechanism, it can frequently serve the individual well in preventing overwhelming anxiety or marked depression."[7]

Often, however, denial is not healthy. In fact, it may ignore or distort reality.

The first time denial might come into play for the cancer patient is before diagnosis. He has a symptom he knows to be one of the warning signs of cancer, but he denies it and does not seek medical care.

When diagnosis is finally made, denial is put to work again. "There must have been some mistake," says the patient. "Maybe the laboratory got the names mixed up." The patient may go from doctor to doctor in an effort to disprove the diagnosis.

As the disease progresses, all of the negative information is minimized, and the positive information is emphasized. Physicians commonly encourage this sort of denial, thinking they must maintain hope as long as possible. But there is a fine line between having a positive attitude and denying reality. It is best to face reality—and to know the truth. Do not pretend cancer does not exist when it does. See the situation as it really is—no worse and no better.

Resenting help. Betty Olsen, the mother of three active preschoolers at the time of diagnosis, enjoyed her busy routine of caring for the children, cleaning, cooking, gardening and canning. She took pride in doing things herself.

The diagnosis of uterine cancer did not have much effect on Betty's self-esteem at first.

"I was just so relieved to have the tumor removed," she said, "that I didn't think too much about it. I can remember thinking I was glad, at least, that it was in the uterus instead of the breast. At least the surgery didn't show!

"But I had to go back into the hospital later for a rather vigorous round of therapy, and I had to be away from my husband and kids for three weeks. While I was at the hospital, I kept imagining how terrible it was for them. I had always done everything for everybody—they even needed me to pick out their clothes every day.

"When I got home, I was shocked. Why, it didn't look like they had missed me one bit! I'd never seen the house so clean, and the kids were all making their own beds and picking out their own clothes to wear! I knew I should have been happy about them getting along so well, but I guess my pride was hurt. Instead of being happy, I was really resentful."

Being able to accept help from others is often very difficult for the cancer patient. Knowing he *needs* help adds to his feelings of helplessness and vulnerability.

The problem of accepting help is tied strongly to the patient's intense desire to be "normal" and not be different from anyone else. Because there might be times when he is totally dependent on others to help him, his self-esteem can be badly bruised.

Remembering the patient's fragile self-esteem, family and friends should offer help in a gentle, sensitive way. The patient should be encouraged to do as much as he possibly can.

Self-esteem can be boosted, too, by asking the patient his advice or opinion regarding a problem you might have. People who have suffered difficulties often have great depth of character and can give excellent counsel.

Compensation. A person compensates by counterbalancing his shortcomings with a concentration on his strengths.

This concept is beautifully illustrated by the story of Joni Eareckson Tada who, as an athletic teenager, had a diving accident and became a quadriplegic. Her self-esteem had centered largely on her athletic ability: horseback riding, water skiing, swimming. Her diving accident took away the ability to use her arms and legs.

Eventually, she discovered that her talent for drawing, which she had enjoyed before the accident, was not confined to her useless hands. By learning to draw with a pen in her mouth, she developed this talent amazingly. By *compensating* in this way, she found both a means of expression and a rewarding career.

It is important for any person who has endured physical limitations because of cancer to look for an area that he can develop to compensate for his loss.

Bearing one another's burdens. Another means of maintaining or restoring self-esteem is found in the Christian commandment to "bear one another's burdens." Dr. James Dobson describes the psychological effect of this principle.

> I have repeatedly observed that a person's needs and problems seem less threatening when he is busy helping someone else handle theirs. It is difficult to wallow in your own troubles when you are actively shouldering another person's load and seeking solutions to his problems. For each discouraged reader who feels unloved and shortchanged by life, I would recommend that you consciously make a practice of giving to others. Visit the sick. Bake something for your neighbor. Use your car for those without transportation. And perhaps most importantly, learn to be a good listener. The world is filled with lonely, disheartened people like yourself, and you are in an excellent position to empathize with them. And while you're doing it, I guarantee that your own sense of uselessness will begin to fade. [8]

This concept was put into practice by a woman who, because of massive surgery for cancer, was forced to quit her job of over thirty years. Thinking that she was totally useless, Emma was swallowed up in despair.

"I was not married," she says, "and I had no family. My life revolved around my career. Suddenly my daily routine no longer existed; my financial status changed greatly. This left a feeling of uselessness. I got so depressed I didn't care if I lived or not."

With the help of Nell Collins, a former nurse who has a ministry to cancer patients, Emma slowly began to see God's love and plan for her life. As time went on, she started helping Nell by typing letters and taking care of some other paperwork. As Nell's work expanded, so did her secretarial needs, and a woman who had thought of herself as useless became the "right arm" of a growing service.

We cannot understand our real value in terms of beauty, intelligence, and talent. To see our true worth we must begin to understand the extent of God's love for each of us. Jesus, God's Son, willingly sacrificed his life to bring peace between God and us. His action indicates what God must consider our true worth to be—whether or not we have cancer.

Facing Negative Emotions

Anne Jones, mother of a six-year-old boy, was thirty-two when she discovered a lump in her breast. The biopsy proved the tumor to be malignant, and she immediately had a radical mastectomy of the left side.

"I tried to be really brave at first," she says. "I was going to show everyone how beautifully I could cope—I'd be the model example of courage. I was going to fly through this thing with no problem, just like a breeze.

"I was able to muddle through for a little while before I fell apart. Completely.

"I saw myself as ugly, deformed. I thought that everyone saw my ugliness. When they looked at me, I was sure that was all they saw. I struck out at everyone and everything. I hated everybody. I struck out in words, in visciousness, in bitterness, with a scowl on my face. I was going to make everyone else feel just as miserable as I did."

EXPECT EMOTIONAL STRUGGLES

The cancer patient and those who love him may be discouraged, worried, depressed. There will be days when (fear) is powerful. The cancer patient may have times when the medication he is taking makes him despondent. He probably will feel tremendous resentment that this terrible thing should happen to him.

Some patients may put on a fantastic performance, attempting to gloss over their real feelings so that family members will not be upset. This kind of patient is typically (but not necessarily) a mother who is trying to protect her family.

Other times, family members, too, try to protect the patient from anything unpleasant. The result is usually a great deal of playacting and virtually no communication. The family members deceive themselves into thinking that the patient is handling it "just fine." If negative emotions are not faced squarely, they can become snarled in a web that is nearly impossible to untangle.

Facing a Negative Emotion

1. Identify it.
2. Acknowledge it.
3. See it as God sees it.
4. When it is sin, confess it.
5. Ask God to replace it with a positive emotion.

What are the negative emotions with which the cancer patient may have to contend?

Fear. Every cancer patient experiences a degree of fear. The dictionary calls fear a "painful feeling of impending danger." This emotion wears many disguises: anxiety, doubt, timidity, indecision, superstition, withdrawal, loneliness, overaggression, worry, feelings of inferiority, cowardice, hesitance, depression, haughtiness, shyness.[1]

Sometimes our fear is so great we become afraid of our fear. Eileen Tiedt in *Nursing Forum* describes the process in this manner:

> Individuals respond to fear and anxiety in different ways. They may withdraw, become depressed, become demanding. Fear and a high level of anxiety may be interpreted by the patient to mean he or she is losing emotional control. Loss of self-control is a crucial threat to the integrity of any person; thus, the lack of control, generated by the original fear, increases the fear and a vicious circle ensues.[2]

Some cancer patients find it helpful to memorize Bible verses to repeat when fear strikes them. Elsa, for example, would panic at times when her breath was halted because of her lung cancer. She memorized a few verses, and they helped calm her during frightening moments.

Listed below are some Bible passages to encourage patients and their families in times of fear.

- "God is our refuge and strength, a very present help in trouble. Therefore we will not fear, though the earth should change, and though the mountains slip into the heart of the sea" (Ps. 46:1, 2).
- "When I am afraid, I will put my trust in Thee" (Ps. 56:3).
- "Do not fear, for I have redeemed you; I have called you by name; you are Mine! When you pass through the waters, I will be with you; and through the rivers, they will not overflow you. When you walk through the fire, you will not be scorched, nor will the flame burn you. For I am the Lord your God, the Holy One of Israel, your Savior" (Isa. 43:1-3).
- "For God hath not given us a spirit of fear, but of power and of love and of a sound mind" (2 Tim. 1:7, KJV).

Anger Often cancer patients find themselves angry because they have cancer. The object of anger may be God, because he allowed the illness to occur. "I shook my fist at God and screamed at him!" one cancer patient related.

Anger is manifested in a number of ways: envy, intolerance, criticism, revenge, hatred, rebellion, jealousy, unforgiveness, bitterness, indignation, wrath, quarreling.[3]

Psychologists have found that unresolved anger always plays a part in depression and usually is involved, in some way, in other kinds of mental and emotional illness. Doc-

Fifteen Reasons Cancer Patients Are Afraid

Fear is a normal reaction to the diagnosis of cancer. The fear, sometimes, is of the unknown. A cancer patient might be tortured by the following factors.

He does not know:

1. What caused the cancer;
2. If the surgeon got it all;
3. If he will have to suffer a lot of pain, and if so, if he will be able to handle it;
4. How it will affect his physical appearance;
5. If it has spread (metastasized) to another location in his body;
6. What effect it will have on his children, or if they will become overly worried about their own bodies;
7. If he will be a burden to his family;
8. Which treatment will work best;
9. How his body will react to treatment, or what side effects he might have;
10. How long he will live;
11. If the people around him are telling him the truth, or if they are trying to hide something from him (he is suspicious of everyone);
12. How much money this whole thing will cost;
13. If he will be able to continue to work, or if he will become dependent;
14. If his mate will still love him and stand beside him;
15. What dying is like, or if there is life after death.

tors now see a direct link between anger and many physical illnesses.

In order to resolve anger, a person must first acknowledge that he is angry. Anger that is denied leads in an insidious way to resentment. A person can harbor resentment without being consciously aware that he is doing so. Acknowledging anger and confessing it when it is sin has a remarkable dissipating effect.

Depression. Depression is a common problem in our society. Tranquilizers and antidepressants are sold in huge volumes both legally and illegally—indicating that depression is not a condition limited to the cancer patient. After a few days or weeks, tranquilizers themselves often cause depression.

Watching the evening news is enough to make a person mildly depressed. The world is full of sad, tragic, and miserable circumstances.

Of course, this problem of depression can be caused by a physical abnormality or a chemical or hormonal imbalance. If you are depressed, you should first check with your physician to see if there is a physical cause. Powerful chemotherapy drugs sometimes cause depression, also.

Most depression, however, is mental or emotional in nature. Usually it is the result of unresolved anger or fear with resentment added.

People, in a general sense, tend to be

either anger-prone or fear-prone. One person will respond with anger to a given set of circumstances, while another person will respond with fear to the same set of circumstances. Fear and anger are powerful emotions and, if repressed, naturally lead to a state of depression.

It is important to try to uncover the underlying cause of the depression. Dr. Roy W. Menninger, president of the Menninger Foundation, says, "You can't jolly people out of depression, or shame them out of it. In most people, depression is a kind of repressed anger, and these people have given up any effort to express that anger."[4]

In *How to Win Over Depression*, Tim LaHaye says that sickness itself is one of the major causes of depression.

> Everyone has his breaking point. We have already seen that some people can endure more pressure or depression-producing circumstances than others. But whatever your tolerance for depression, it will be lowered through illness. Protracted periods of illness make you even more vulnerable. . . . In addition, when a person is weakened or debilitated by illness, things that would ordinarily not bother him tend to be unduly magnified. It is probably easier to drift into self-pity during an illness than at any other period.[5]

Severe depression can result in despair. The thought of facing the future with all its uncertainties may seem too much to bear. You, as the patient, may come to the place

Recommended Reading
Tim LaHaye gives a thorough treatment
of depression in his book *How to Win Over
Depression* (Grand Rapids, Mich.: Zondervan, 1974).

where you believe your family would be
better off without you. You might feel it
would be better for everybody if you just
jumped out the window.

Suicide causes family members more terrible grief than any other cause of death.
The very ones you want to protect from the
ordeal of your debilitating illness will suffer
much more if you take your own life. You
will burden them with a heart-wrenching
sense of guilt if you take such action.

If anyone reading this book is experiencing
these feelings, I urge you to look to God for
the answer to your depression. He can give
you hope; he can meet each of your needs.

Doubt. Illness may lead cancer patients
to question things they had taken for granted
before, including spiritual beliefs. Does God
exist? Does he love me? How could he let
this happen? Is Christ the only way to God?

God welcomes honest searching. Chris-
tianity is based on historical fact, not on the
speculations of men. It will not collapse
under close examination. The cancer patient
should ask questions. Seek answers. Talk to
God about doubts and questions. Search the
Bible for answers. The Scriptures address

doubts and questions. Its answers may lead a person to a new level of commitment.

Worry Worry eats away at your heart, mind, and spirit. It damages your sense of well-being. Worry is a handmaiden to cancer; so many things are not known; so many tests have to be run; it takes so long to get the results.

Cancer causes a mother to worry about who will take care of the children while she is ill, or if she should die. Cancer causes anxiety about physical appearance. Mastectomy patients especially worry about how their husbands will react to the results of breast surgery.

Every cancer patient hopes he will be cured, but the worry that the cancer will someday return never goes away. Money is an enormous worry, especially if insurance is inadequate. Cancer care is expensive, and worry about money can plague not only the cancer patient but everyone in the family.

Worry can destroy a person. But the Bible offers an alternative.

Don't worry about anything; instead, pray about everything; tell God your needs and don't forget to thank him for his answers. If you do this you will experience God's peace, which is far more wonderful than the human mind can understand. His peace will keep your thoughts and your hearts quiet and at rest as you trust in Christ Jesus (Phil. 4:6, 7, TLB).

Regret or remorse. "If only I had gone to the doctor sooner."

"Why did I say those mean things to him? I should have known he was sick."

"If only . . . if only . . . if only. . . ."

Regret is a wasted emotion. It is futile; in no way can it change things. What is done is done, and no amount of self-recrimination can change the past. Regret and remorse are guilt feelings in disguise. If not resolved, these feelings also lead to depression.

Sometimes regret is more of a problem for the family members than it is for the cancer patient. A mother may torture herself with real or imagined failings and in the end blame herself for her child's sickness. This is agony beyond belief, and it is not necessary.

Of course, we make mistakes, and some of those mistakes have heavy consequences. Just remember: you did the very best you could with the information you had at the time.

You can become totally preoccupied with regret. If you have done or said something wrong, confess it to God and *accept his forgiveness*.

RECOGNIZE SPIRITUAL NEEDS

Sometimes negative emotions are symptoms of spiritual needs. Nell Collins conducts a seminar for nurses on the subject "How to Recognize a Spiritual Need." The following are the most easily recognized symptoms.

1. *Rejection of people.* Often a patient will turn his face to the wall and refuse to communicate with anybody. Sometimes this is because his visitor refuses to talk about spiritual matters, and the patient does not want to talk about anything else.

2. *Tears.* Though tears can be a sign of many other feelings, such as worry, anxiety, or loneliness, it is possible the patient is distraught because he feels he does not have the right relationship with God.

3. *Floor-pacing.* This person is often quite sleepy, but he cannot sleep because he has a spiritual need that is not being met. So he walks the floor.

4. *Change in normal sleep patterns.* A spiritual need could be expressed by a radical change in sleep patterns. Either inability to sleep (insomnia) or sleeping far more than normal is a danger signal.

5. *Open admission of fear.* A patient might readily admit he is afraid.

6. *Despondence.* No matter how much wealth or success has been realized in life, a person will feel distressed until he has had his spiritual needs met.

7. *Egocentric trip.* The only person this patient can talk about is himself. The pro-

nouns *I, me,* and *my* are prominent in his conversation.

8. *Spiritual introversion.* This person refuses to talk to his church leader or anyone else about spiritual matters. A spiritual withdrawing often looks as if the patient does not want to discuss these things; often the reverse is true.

HOW TO HELP MEET SOMEONE'S SPIRITUAL NEEDS

Once the spiritual needs have been recognized, you can begin to help the patient. The following guidelines can direct your efforts.

Make sure that you yourself are not confused about the meaning of death and possibly even your own relationship with God. If you are not sure of your own beliefs, you should direct the patient to some other person who can help. Ask if he wants a visit from the pastor of a Bible-believing church.

Listen to the patient. This is probably the most helpful thing you can do. The cancer patient will be frustrated if you will not let him talk about his fears. Even if the prognosis is good, he may want to talk about the possibility of death. Let him talk, and do not be patronizing ("Now, now, you don't need to be worrying about *that*"). If the prognosis is poor, the family may be so concerned with "How are we going to tell him?" that they fail to hear when the patient tells *them* that he is dying.

Let the patient talk about death if he wants

to. If you cringe and refuse to talk, or if you change the subject every time he mentions it, you might as well be saying that it is too horrible to even suggest. That attitude is not helpful.

Remember the importance of hope. It is good to hope that the chemotherapy will work, to hope that the radiation therapy will be effective, to hope that the third surgery will take care of the cancer. It is also good to hope that research will find a new cure for the kind of cancer he has.

Many patients maintain to the very end some kind of hope that the physical condition will improve. The patient should not be made to feel that he has been "given up."

On the other hand, the family should be sensitive to the fact that the patient's hopes will change as he begins accepting the reality of his situation. It will only frustrate the patient for you to keep talking about hopes he recognizes to be no longer valid.

Recognize the difference between temporary hope and ultimate hope. Ultimate hope is hope in God. It will give complete peace. Chapter 5 can help you and your friend or loved one attain that ultimate hope.

The Hopeful Side of Death

Today there is tremendous interest in the subject of death and the process of dying. The public is bombarded with books, articles, and television talkshows that probe the subject. Colleges and universities all over the country have added courses on dying. People can discuss death with doctors, nurses, psychiatrists, and chaplains.

But still too often even in our "enlightened" age, people face the end of their own lives with too little preparation, too little opportunity to talk openly, and too much pretending.

BREAKING THE SILENCE BARRIER

Generally, doctors have been taught to treat illness. They see death as the ultimate enemy and fight that enemy vigorously and courageously. To many doctors, however, death means failure, and some, sadly, find it difficult themselves to face the reality of death.

The patient is often the one who must set the tone as far as frankness is concerned. Tell your doctor you want to know everything, if you do. Tell the members of your family that you want to talk about dying, if you want silence about it broken. You may need to be insistent, because they might be reluctant to discuss it.

If *you* do not bring up the subject, however, they will probably be afraid to mention it. The more open and candid you are, the more honest they will be able to be. Great tension can be relieved by opening those lines of communication.

WHAT ABOUT THE FUTURE?

The following suggestions can help a cancer patient prepare for the days to come. They can also serve as the basis for honest talks with close friends and family members.

Cherish life. Dying is a part of life. Each of us is one day closer to his own death today than he was yesterday. Each day is very precious, and we should not waste our remaining time being miserable about the fact that this life must come to an end.

Live each day to the full. No one knows how long he will live; no one can be sure what tomorrow will bring. But one does need to live each day to the full, even if he is confined to bed.

One lovely Christian woman could not get up from her bed, but she blessed hundreds of people by telephoning shut-ins and writing cheerful notes of comfort to those in need. People who are confined by illness or infirmity can pray for others.

Daily Confidence Builders

1. Start the day with God. Pray and read a portion of the Bible.
2. Define your physical capabilities for the day.
3. Set realistic but worthy goals. Write them on paper in order of priority.
4. Make an honest attempt to meet your goals, even if you don't feel like it.
5. Be involved with people when at all possible. Serve *their* needs.

Accept the grieving process. It is not unusual or wrong to grieve about losing a loved one or one's own life. Family members grieve because they are losing a person they love. The dying person grieves because he is losing *everyone* he loves in this world. A person who has chosen to follow Christ will grieve, but he has the hope of an eternal life. He can cling to the wonderful promise of being reunited with his believing relatives and friends in heaven.

Draw close to your family. Families who have close relationships before the onset of a serious illness seem to bear the distress of a terminal illness better than families who have not been as close. Sometimes members withdraw from a cancer patient. They seem unable to communicate because of their own fear and misery. They may feel guilty about past failures and conflicts with the patient. Other times patients feel guilty because they have to rely on others for their needs. One person said she felt bad about "causing so much trouble for my family."

Despite these obstacles, communication within a family can take place during this time, perhaps in a way not possible ordinarily. Do not hesitate to be the one to initiate the mending of broken or faltering relationships.

Guard against loneliness. Profound loneliness is often one of the most intense feelings of the dying patient. Family members and friends often stay away because they do not know what to say, but frequent visits are of prime importance at a time like this.

Cicely Saunders, an authority on treatment of the terminally ill, reports: "A dying patient needs above all someone to listen and understand how he feels. Those who stay away from these patients because they feel they can bring nothing but their lack of understanding should realize that it is our desire to *try* to understand, and not our success in doing so, that eases the loneliness that is so hard to bear."[1]

Build your faith. It is interesting also that Saunders says patients with a strong religious faith were least anxious, while those with tepid faith were more anxious than those with none. She notes that there is a great difference between "intrinsic" and "extrinsic" religion. "Those who think of religion as a sort of insurance against trouble do not find such a belief sustaining in adversity, although they sometimes find a more mature faith when they are dying."[2]

HANDLING PHYSICAL PAIN

One of the strongest fears associated with the word *cancer* is that the disease will inevitably cause severe and untreatable pain. Cicely Saunders states in *Nursing Times* that this misconception can cause needless suffering.

"People live in fear of the onset of pain," she says, "and, if it occurs, because it is thought to be inevitable, no complaint is made and no relief given. As a district nurse said sadly to us on a day visit, 'They don't know how much pain they are supposed to have.' "

She goes on to explain that 50 percent of those persons who die from all forms of malignant disease should experience no pain at all. Another 10 percent may be expected to have mild pain only. The more severe pain experienced by the remainder "can be abolished while the patient still remains alert, able to enjoy the company of those around him and often able to be up and about until near his death."[3]

She maintains that "successful treatment may call for much imagination and persistence."[4] If you are encountering severe pain that is not being controlled by your medication, you might suggest to your physician that you would like to be seen by a doctor who specializes in this area. Most doctors are glad to have a consultation and want very much for you to be as comfortable as possible.

WHEN DEATH BECOMES PERSONAL

Whether a person plans to die at home, in a hospital, or hospice, or somewhere else, he must face the reality of his own death.

To a dying person, death is no longer the subject of abstract philosophical debate. It is real, imminent, and it is personal.

People have pondered death throughout the ages. All kinds of ideas and theories have been proposed. Archaeology has confirmed that people in every culture and civilization have believed in a supernatural power, and that there is a universal belief that man's spirit does not die with the body.

Today many false theories about what happens after death are popular. How do we know these theories are false? God has given us a divine yardstick by which we can evaluate any theory. That yardstick is the Bible. If a theory goes against Scripture, it has to be false.

FOUR FALSEHOODS ABOUT
THE AFTERLIFE

No hereafter. This life is all we have, some say. Everything we shall ever have is right here on earth. This theory is popularly sup-

An Alternative:
The Hospice Movement

Treatment of the severe pain sometimes felt by terminally ill patients has been one of the major concerns of the hospice movement. The word *hospice* means "way station," and it is a facility, something between a hospital and a home, where terminally ill patients can receive the special care they need. Regular hospital routines, geared to saving lives and curing illnesses, in many cases have not met the needs of the terminally ill.

The hospice movement is really nothing new. Peoples in various cultures in both ancient and modern times have been concerned with the care of the dying. The modern hospice movement began in England. Today new hospices are being formed in cities all over this country.

The hospice usually is a place where family members can be trained to care for the terminally ill at home. Most patients want to be at home with their families as much as possible. If, however, the patient needs more care than can be given at home, he can become an inpatient in the hospice.

Hospice personnel are generally dedicated to relieving pain and making patients feel cared for in a homey atmosphere, while still treating the disease as vigorously as possible. If you are interested in hospice care, call your local hospital. Personnel there should know where the nearest hospice facility is located.

ported by commercials ("You only go around once") and familiar songs like "I'm gonna live 'til I die."

Annihilation of the wicked. The good live forever, it is said, but the wicked become nonexistent. This theory is popularly supported at funerals where emphasis is placed on how "good" the person was. "He was a good man," acquaintances say, implying that his goodness will earn him passage to heaven. The "bad" people, on the other hand, are simply blotted out.

Transmigration of the soul. The theory that the spirit of man goes on to live in another body is called "transmigration of the soul." This theory is often seen in the occult and Eastern religions, and is the basis for theories of reincarnation.

Universal salvation. Today the most popular theory of all is based on the fact of God's perfect love; his perfect *justice* is forgotten. God is love, it is said, and a loving God wouldn't condemn anyone, would he?

These theories, interesting as they are, are false because they conflict with Scripture. They are dangerous, too, because they give people a false sense of security.

WHAT THE BIBLE SAYS ABOUT DEATH

The Bible teaches that the human spirit does not die. "And the Lord God formed man of the dust of the ground, and breathed into his nostrils the breath of life; and *man became a living soul*" (Gen. 2:7, KJV).

God created man perfect and eternal, and though sin destroyed man's perfection, his spirit remains eternal.

Because of God's holiness, sinful man *cannot* spend eternity with him. To permit this would be totally inconsistent with God's holy nature. Therefore, whoever sins is *alienated* from God during his physical life and separated from God throughout eternity. This state is called "spiritual death."

Every one of us deserves to experience spiritual death, because not one of us can meet God's standards of perfection. "For all have sinned, and come short of the glory of God" (Rom. 3:23, KJV).

The good news is that God loved us so much he sent his Son to die for us and to pay the penalty for our sins.

When a person trusts Jesus Christ to be his own Savior, he is "born again." This spiritual birth transfers him from the state of spiritual death into the state of spiritual life. God himself comes to live in that believer in the person of the Holy Spirit. Consequently a Christian can know (not hope) that if he should die, he would immediately be with Christ (2 Cor. 5:8).

THE TRUTH ABOUT HEAVEN

What lies beyond the grave for a believer?

Joseph Bayly, a man who saw three of

his sons die, wrote about heaven in *The View from a Hearse:*

> I cannot prove the existence of heaven. I accept its reality by faith, on the authority of Jesus Christ: "In my Father's house are many mansions: if it were not so, I would have told you. I go to prepare a place for you."
>
> For that matter, if I were a twin in the womb, I doubt that I could prove the existence of earth to my mate. He would probably object that the idea of an earth beyond the womb was ridiculous, that the womb was the only earth we'd ever know.
>
> If I tried to explain that earthlings live in a greatly expanded environment and breathe air, he would only be more skeptical. After all, a fetus lives in water; who could imagine its being able to live in a universe of air? To him such a transition would seem impossible.
>
> It would take birth to prove the earth's existence to a fetus. A little pain, a dark tunnel, a gasp of air—and then the wide world! Green grass, laps, lakes, the ocean, horses (could a fetus imagine a horse?), rainbows, walking, running, surfing, ice-skating. With enough room that you don't have to shove, and a universe beyond.[5]

Like the fetus, we cannot envision what it will be like on the other side of the tunnel—in heaven. But from the Bible, God's Word, we can know this much:

- Heaven is a place of rest (Rev. 14:13).
- Heaven is a place without pain, weeping, or mourning (Rev. 21:4).

- Heaven is a place of total joy in the presence of the Lord (Acts 2:28).
- Though we will be changed, we will recognize our loved ones (Matt. 17:3, 4; Peter recognized Moses and Elijah).
- Heaven will be more beautiful than anything we can imagine (Rev. 21-22).
- We will be comfortable in heaven, for it will be *home* (John 14:2).

CHAPTER 6

Ten Questions Families Ask

Cancer does not strike in a vacuum. Not only is the patient affected, but also every member of the family: children, parents, brothers, sisters, husband, or wife. The relationships of the family members are all put under severe stress.

If the outlook is good, and surgery has not made a radical change in body image or function, family problems are naturally lessened. The more problems and complications accompanying the cancer, the more traumatic it is for everyone concerned.

A diagnosis of cancer brings many questions from all family members. Questions concerning the medical aspects of the disease should be asked of the physician in charge of the case. Write out a list before you see your doctor so you can be sure every question is answered. Remember, however, that some questions cannot be answered. If he does not know, the doctor will say so.

The following questions are the ones I have heard most frequently from families of cancer patients. I have talked with doctors, nurses, patients, and family members to find answers.

Should small children be told that a parent has cancer?

Children have an amazing capacity to deal with truth. They will be hurt far more in the long run if you try to keep the illness a secret from them. If they do not find out from you, they will hear from someone else. Whispers and huddled conferences cause children more alarm than does the truth.

Of course, the *way* you tell them is extremely important. It will do them no good for you to be overly emotional, hysterical, or in a state of despair. It might be best to ask the doctor to explain what is happening in a medical sense if you are too upset to do so.

If the children are quite young, you might tell them something like this: "Mommy found that she had something growing in her body that wasn't supposed to be there. It is called a tumor. The doctors had to remove the tumor, because it was very dangerous for it to be there. The tumor is sometimes called *cancer.* This is a very scary word, because sometimes people die when they have this kind of tumor growing in their bodies. Doctors now know a great deal more than they used to about taking care of people who have this happen." If the prognosis is good, say, "We think Mommy is going to be just fine."

Children should be given some specific information about the particular medical treatment, but should not be overburdened with too many details. They should be told the truth in a matter-of-fact manner. Above all, do not lie to the children. Do not tell them Mommy has the flu or some other minor problem. Tell them the doctors are doing everything they can. Do not be afraid to say, "I don't know."

If the disease gets progressively worse, tell the children that Mommy might not be able to get well. Reassure them that they will be loved, cared for, and not abandoned. Listen carefully to the questions they ask, and answer as simply and honestly as you can.

What if the parent dies?

If the parent should die, it is important that the child be allowed to grieve. This may seem obvious, but often in the midst of their own grief, family members will say things like, "You must be a big, brave boy now." This makes the child feel he cannot show emotion, so he keeps it all bottled up inside. Let him know it is all right for him to feel sad and to miss his parent.

Children often feel a tremendous sense of guilt because of the death of a parent. If the parent was ill at home, the child was probably told to keep quiet so the parent could rest. If the parent then dies, the child might conclude that he was not quiet enough, that he was responsible for the death. Help the child to openly discuss these fears and guilt feelings.

One little girl might be saddled for life with guilt feelings about her mother's death. Her mother, Dorothy, just was not feeling well, but nothing very specific seemed to be wrong. At last Dorothy went to the hospital for tests. Diagnosis: cancer of the liver. She died within three weeks.

Her little girl was six years old. An aunt came to stay with her while her mother was in the hospital. The aunt repeatedly said to others in front of the child, "Dorothy never had any problems until *that* girl was born." It is highly unlikely that the cancer had any connection whatsoever with the birth of the little girl six years before, and no one knows what caused the aunt to reach this conclusion. The point, however, is that the child heard these remarks and very likely believed herself responsible for her mother's death.

Be very careful what you say when tender little ones are around—even when you think they are not listening.

Should children go to the funeral of a parent?

I believe children over three years of age should be permitted to attend the funeral and burial of a loved one. It is hard if the child's first encounter with death is that of a parent, but he needs to be included in these ceremonies. The experience of the funeral is important in helping the living, including children, come to terms with the fact of death.

"I feel very blessed," said one young mother to me just a few weeks before she died. "I'm so glad I can talk about my death with my children. I can tell them that when they see my body at the funeral home, they'll be seeing just the shell. The 'real me' will not be there. The real me will be with Jesus. And, someday, when God says the time is right, we'll be reunited in that wonderful place! Isn't that great? If I had died suddenly in a car accident or something, we'd never have had these precious times together."

What about parents of grown children who have cancer? What should their role be?

Parents of an adult with cancer can be a blessing—or a cause for stress.

Be available; be sensitive. Offer help in a way so that your grown child can maintain self-esteem. Do not make him or her feel incapable. If there are young children needing care, grandparents can be a great help.

Be extra sensitive to the needs of your child's husband or wife. You may have to step aside and let the spouse make decisions you feel entitled to make. You may not agree with every decision the spouse makes; but it is, nevertheless, his or her decision.

Mothers can sometimes tremendously upset grown daughters who have cancer by hovering and being emotionally distraught.

The daughter then feels guilty about causing her mother so much grief. Also, the daughter can see right through it if the mother is putting up a front. The mother's visits should not be extremely long while her daughter is in the hospital recovering from surgery, because they might be emotionally tiring for her.

I feel I should be at the hospital every minute. If I have something come up that keeps me from visiting, I feel terribly guilty. What about this?

It is important for close family members to keep a balance during the time when their loved one is hospitalized and confined. You will want to be there as much as possible, yet you cannot become a slave to your own imagination about what you should or should not do. Very few people are so free from obligations that they can live in the hospital with the patient. All you can do is your best. Do not expect more of yourself.

Other people besides the patient need you. Your work needs you. You need you. Do not let a tyrannical sense of martyrdom obsess you. Do all that you possibly can, and let others help. If you have a church home, tell your pastor about your needs and limitations.

The patient may not feel like having a constant stream of visitors, anyway. That might be tiring. Ask the patient how he feels about visitors. It may be that he would like some time alone. On the other hand, too little visiting can make the patient feel abandoned, alone, and very depressed.

It is so hard to know what to say during a visit. What should a visitor say or not say when visiting a cancer patient in the hospital?

Making conversation is sometimes extremely difficult, especially if the patient is depressed and anxious. You know that he does not want to talk about the weather any more than you do.

Here are some suggestions, however.

1. Do not tell the patient how "lucky" he is. He does not feel one bit lucky.

2. Do not tell him how great he looks, unless he really does. You can pick out something that actually does look good, for example, "Your color looks much better today." Or, "You look like you had a good night's rest."

3. Super-happy and bouncy visitors may make the patient feel worse. Take it easy until you see how he is feeling.

4. Do not tell him what a rough week you have had.

5. Do not tell him that you know just how he feels. You do not.

6. Do ask him if he feels like talking. Be an active listener. Encourage him to express himself to you.

7. He might like you to read to him some words of comfort from the Bible. Paul wrote

the book of Philippians while in prison, yet the book is overflowing with joy. That might be a good place to read.

8. Go into the room with a warm smile and say hi. A hug or pat on the arm can express much of what you want to say. You can find out what is on the patient's mind by saying something like, "How are you handling it?"

9. The sense of touch is extremely important, especially when a person is in the midst of trauma. Very often people recoil from the cancer patient, standing back from the bed, refusing to touch him, giving the impression that the diagnosis might be leprosy. *Cancer is not contagious.* Hold the patient's hand and sit on the side of the bed if it is comfortable for him. Your physical closeness will be solacing.

What kind of emotional responses might the cancer patient have?

One of the greatest problems of family members is dealing with the emotional upset of the cancer patient when they are also traumatized.

You might as well expect the cancer patient to exhibit any or all of these emotional responses: anger, fear, depression, irritability, sleeplessness, and bizarre dreams. Increased sexual feelings often are part of unusual tension and stress, and the patient may feel guilty because of these feelings. If he or she does not know how to handle guilt, that will add to the anxiety.

A special problem for men experiencing the progressively debilitating process of terminal cancer is the sense of a "loss of manliness." This problem causes depression, which may be expressed in hostility toward the family, especially the wife.

What special problems face the family when the condition is terminal and in the last stages, and the patient is being cared for at home?

Families who choose to care for a terminally ill patient at home usually are glad afterward that they have done so. It is a stressful time, but many families grow very close and find unforeseen blessings in such a situation.

The word *terminal* sometimes suggests to people that nothing more can be done for the patient. This is not true. It may be that nothing more can be done to cure the cancer, but there is always much that can be done to make the patient more comfortable.

The primary caretaker will not be able to manage all the bedside nursing responsibilities. Bathing, feeding, changing dressings, changing sheets, changing the patient's position, relieving constipation, and sitting up at night are just a few of the many important things to be done. Frequent rubdowns of back, buttocks, elbows, heels, and knees also make the patient more comfortable. A comfortable, dry bed is as essential as loving, compassionate nursing care. If you are not the primary caretaker, offer to help in any way you can.

About half of the people who die from cancer experience no pain at all from the disease, and powerful pain medication is available for those who do. Visiting nurses can sometimes come to your home and help you with specific problems regarding pain, feeding, and so forth.

Most families in this situation need some sort of special equipment—hospital beds, walkers, wheelchairs. This kind of equipment is usually available on a rental or loan basis. Call your local chapter of the American Cancer Society; the ACS will direct you to someone who can help. Your local public health department can advise you as to the availability of visiting nurses, and many chapters of the Veterans of Foreign Wars lend wheelchairs and other equipment.

Inability to sleep is another commonly encountered problem for family members, and this problem adds to the emotional stress of the situation. The ability to cope is directly related to being rested. A family member may need to see the doctor to get medical help for insomnia. *You must get adequate sleep.*

Trying to maintain normal family activities during a time such as this is nearly impossible. Ask for help. If you are an extremely capable person, members of the extended family may not know that you need help. Explain your needs specifically. If you do not have an extended family, your church family will help if the pastor is made aware of your needs.

I find that I am depending on our physician for emotional support and am usually disappointed. What should I expect from him?

Family members and the patient tend to look to the physician for emotional support on an ongoing basis, particularly in the last stages. Most people express the desire for the physician to give more emotional support and to take more time to explain what is happening. Some physicians give this kind of emotional support, and some do not.

Families and patients often endow the physician with superhuman qualities, then are disappointed to find he is only human. Most physicians working with cancer patients are extremely knowledgeable and concerned. But they are just human beings with limited knowledge doing the best they can. It is really not fair to expect them to be more than that.

What about financial problems?

Cancer costs can be overwhelming, but help is available. The ACS reports: "Individuals have several sources of help in paying for cancer costs," including third-party payers such as Blue Cross and private insurance companies, public agencies, and private health organizations. Cancer is covered by personal insurance plans either under narrowly defined cancer policies or through catastrophic illness provisions in comprehensive insurance programs.

"Hospital costs," the ACS reminds us,

"can be reduced by using nursing facilities, hospices for advanced cancer patients, and home care with periodic professional medical visits."

Any family encountering cancer should take advantage of the financial counseling usually offered through the hospital social workers. Review your insurance policies to make sure you understand and receive all the benefits to which you are entitled. Many drugs can be provided free by the National Cancer Institute. Check with your county welfare agency and Social Security office to see if you would be eligible for Medicare or Medicaid benefits.

Children with Cancer

In an address delivered in 1977, C. Everett Koop, M.D., then Surgeon-in-Chief of the Children's Hospital of Philadelphia, stated, "The diagnosis of cancer in a child is not only difficult to believe; it is unthinkable."

In the 1950s, victims of childhood leukemia and other cancers were given little hope. The main concern, then, was to make the child as comfortable as possible during his last weeks or months.

While no absolute cure has yet been found, and cancer is second only to accidents as a cause of death in childhood, medical science has made great advances in the treatment of these diseases. More and more patients can hope for full recovery.

These hopes indeed give comfort to the child and the family, but at the same time, the months and even years of intense treatment cause the entire family unit to experience great stress. Death is still a real enemy, and the war against that enemy is often painful, usually financially staggering, and always emotionally draining.

WHAT PARENTS SHOULD EXPECT

James Whitcomb Riley Hospital for children in Indianapolis is, among other things, a treatment center for childhood cancer. The staff of the division of hematology/oncology makes a serious effort to help families and cancer patients face certain problems and circumstances that often accompany the treatment of childhood cancer. Following are some of the problems the staff encounters most often.

Feelings of guilt. The first emotional response seen in the parents is an enormous sense of guilt. Arthur Provisor, M.D., assistant professor of pediatrics in the division of hematology/oncology at Riley, stated in an interview: "Often the early symptoms are very vague, and it's difficult for physicians out in practice to diagnose the problem. These diseases are rather rare, and the early symptoms often resemble other childhood illnesses. Even professionals often do not recognize these early symptoms, so parents should not feel guilty."

Another kind of guilt revolves around the parent-child relationships. Under stress, any parent will probably feel guilty about past failures, both real and imagined. The diagnosis of cancer in the child magnifies the sense of guilt.

A tendency toward overprotection. Parents of a child with cancer will inevitably be overprotective. While the parents know their child has an illness that may take his life, the natural, human reaction is to try to protect that child from any further harm. The result, unhappily, is a life that is anything but normal for the child.

Decisions about activity must be made on an individual basis, but in general the child should go back to school as soon as he is able. He should play with other children. Brothers and sisters should be allowed to have friends over to visit. The parents should feel free to leave him with a baby-sitter. Family vacations and out-of-state travels should not be discontinued if the child is doing well.

Negative response from others. Parents need to be warned that other relatives and family friends may have surprisingly negative reactions. For example, one parent found that her baby-sitter would no longer stay with the children, and some friends refused to come into the house. Even though cancer is not contagious, some people think it is. The parents suddenly have to deal with other people's fears as well as their own.

Parents may need to go to the child's school and explain the disease, the treatment, and the side effects, so the children and teachers will be able to treat the child as normally as possible.

The need for professional care. Parents are often overwhelmed by a sense of being incapable of caring for their child. Pam Flummerfelt, R.N., nurse/clinician and coordinator for the division of hematology/oncology at Riley Hospital for Children, says,

"Staff members need to be sensitive to the fact that the parents have always taken care of this child. Now suddenly, all these other people are taking care of him, and the parent doesn't know how to do some of the things that need to be done. We try to teach the parents to participate in the care of the child. It is comforting to the child, and the parents don't feel left out."

New experiences. Children who are diagnosed with cancer are suddenly faced with many new experiences: frightened parents, serious-faced strangers, a hospital bed, tubes, machines, equipment, and needles. He must face procedures and treatments that either hurt or make him nauseated. Usually the child has never been seriously ill before. He may be scared.

Physical changes. The child and his parents should be prepared for a possible physical change. Very often children under treatment for cancer lose their hair, and frequently the chemotherapy causes a puffiness of the face and abdomen. Children should know in advance that these changes might take place, but that the hair should grow back and the puffiness will go away.

Possible complications. The child with leukemia or other forms of childhood cancer always risks developing serious complications from the therapy. The treatment for the disease may go very well, but other problems, such as hemorrhage or infection, may arise and become very grave.

DISCIPLINING THE SICK CHILD

Often a father and mother will disagree about when, if, and how to discipline their child. If the disagreement is compounded by the knowledge that a child has cancer, the family relationships suffer.

Parents must communicate with each other, decide what behavior is reasonable to expect, then support each other in carrying it out. Part of treating a child "normally" involves discipline. Many parents become extremely lax when their child is sick, and that is not emotionally healthy for the child.

Every child, even a sick child, needs limits set and enforced. A child being sick does not mean he will no longer be willful, disobedient, or rebellious. Any child, sick or not, will test the limits to see if they will be enforced. For the child's sense of security, it is important to set reasonable limits and then make certain that he is lovingly kept within those limits.

In setting limits, however, the parents need to be flexible enough to adjust to changing situations. The treatment for cancer is often painful and stress-producing. The child is undergoing treatments that may cause his behavior to change. He may respond to the treatments with anger, resentment, bitterness, and jealousy of those who are well. These negative emotions, in turn, can cause unacceptable behavior.

The parent needs to be understanding and kind. The child will not understand these powerful negative emotions and will feel guilty about having them. He may not even be able to identify them. The parent must help him understand why he feels the way he does, perhaps by expressing in words what the child is feeling. ("You are feeling angry because you want to be well. You wish you could be well again.")

The parent can help a child express his negative emotions in this manner. Often a torrent of emotions will then pour out, like water from a crumbling dam. Allow the child to express himself. Do not be shocked at his feelings. These feelings need to be expressed, and a sensitive parent can be of tremendous help to a child in this area.

TELLING YOUR CHILD THE TRUTH

Children who are old enough to understand must be told the truth about their disease. One of the most difficult times for the parents is telling the child he has cancer or leukemia, but it is vital that those words be used, even with very young children. If you try to hide the truth from the child, he will not be able to come to terms with his illness; he will fantasize about what is wrong.

If you do not tell him, he will find out sooner or later, and his trust in you will be damaged. Usually hospital staff members help parents over this hurdle by using the words in a matter-of-fact manner during treatment at the time of diagnosis.

A Sample Conversation

When one six-year-old was diagnosed with non-Hodgkins lymphoma, the conversation went something like this:

Dr. A.: "Do you know why you are here, Robert?"

Robert: "No."

Dr. A.: "Would you like to know what's wrong with you?"

Robert: "Yes."

Dr. A.: "Robert, you have a disease called *cancer.* Have you ever known anyone who had cancer?"

Robert: "No."

Dr. A.: "Your body is made up of many cells. When you cut yourself or hurt yourself, the cells may be injured, so some body cells divide to repair the injury.

"However, with cancer, the cells divide without a need, and then you have extra cells. So we will give you treatments to try to stop the cells from dividing. [Dr. A. then drew a diagram to show Robert how the cells divide.]

"Sometimes people are frightened of cancer because they have heard of people who died from cancer, but you don't need to be afraid, because we will try to make you better."

TALKING TO YOUR CHILD ABOUT CANCER

How the truth is told is important. Give the child the facts in a loving, gentle way. Many questions will come up during the course of treatment. Answer them as simply and honestly as possible.

It is not necessary to dwell on the fact of the illness or to talk about it all the time. To do so would make a miserable and far-from-normal situation.

If the time should come that your child's prognosis is poor, you must share that with him. Do not take away all hope for finding a medicine that might help, but acknowledge that he may not be able to get well. He probably knows it anyway, but if you can talk about it, he will not have to bear this knowledge alone.

A mother told me that one of her most meaningful memories was of the day she told her son that he might not recover from his leukemia.

"Do you mean that I'm going to die?" he asked her.

"I don't know the answer to that, Son. But it is possible."

Then they both cried.

Later he told her, "Thanks, Mom. It's good to have someone to cry with."

UNDERSTANDING A CHILD'S FEARS

Sometimes a child fears he has done something bad that caused the cancer. One little boy had heard on television that smoking causes cancer. He was convinced that he had the disease because he had sneaked a couple of his father's cigarettes and smoked them. Other children may feel they are being

Recommended Reading

An excellent book for children with leukemia is *You and Leukemia: A Day at a Time* by Lynn S. Baker. Written for children, it is extremely informative for parents, too. Copies can be obtained by writing to the Mayo Comprehensive Cancer Center, Rochester, Minnesota 55901.

"punished" for times they have misbehaved. Reassure them that this is not the case.

Children of different ages have varying kinds of fears about death. The preschooler may not understand the finality of death, but the school-age child will. Most youngsters are open, honest, and eager to have specific information about what heaven might be like.

A fear common to many children stems from associating death with the word *sleep*. Perhaps when his grandfather died, the child was told, Grandpa is sleeping. He also may have heard of someone dying in his sleep. Because of that, the child may be afraid to sleep or afraid for you to sleep. Discuss with him the use of the word *sleep* and assure him that it is safe to sleep.

A great fear concerning death is the fear of separation from loved ones. Emphasize to the child that Jesus is his very best friend, and he will be with him always, no matter what happens. This truth will help the child deal with his greatest fear: fear of the unknown.

ASSURING BROTHERS AND SISTERS

A child with cancer usually has brothers and/or sisters. These children, too, need information to help them deal with this situation.

Because of the nature of the disease, childhood cancer is usually a long-term problem, having both crisis times and back-to-normal times. Both younger children and older children need to know what is happening. If they are not told that Johnny has a serious problem, they will not understand why he is getting so much attention. They need to be assured that Mommy and Daddy love them just as much as they do Johnny.

A small child needs to be told the truth, gently and sensitively, in language he can understand.

Perhaps he could be told something like this (with the information adjusted to fit the situation): "Johnny has something seriously wrong with his blood. It is called leukemia. This can be a very dangerous disease, and children sometimes die from it. We expect Johnny will live for a long, long time, but we must do everything we can to help him.

"Johnny will be having treatments at the hospital. These are very important to help him get better. Sometimes he will be very sick, and sometimes he will feel just fine. He will be getting a lot of attention. We want you to know that we love you just as much as Johnny, even though we might have to spend a lot more time with him for a while."

Children are truly amazing in the way they rally when the truth is made clear. A brother or sister of a leukemia victim, for example, might willingly go through the pain and trauma of being the donor for a bone marrow transplant. Give each child the opportunity to be part of the family in a meaningful way during this difficult time.

If the prognosis becomes very poor, and death draws near, the siblings should know ahead of time so that they are not caught unprepared for it.

I believe both younger and older siblings should be allowed to attend funeral services. The funeral provides the opportunity to see that the loved one is dead and is not coming back.

"Children are killed every day in automobile accidents," says one mother. "We can't spend the time we have together worrying about when it will end. Life is too precious. We simply have to live while we can, for all of our sakes. I know that my child has cancer, and I know that he may die from it. But we're going to live from day to day. That makes every day very special."

Fifteen Common
Sites of Cancer

There are more than 150 recognizable kinds of cancer. For convenience, cancers are usually grouped according to the part of the body in which the tumor first starts growing.[1]

CANCER OF THE SKIN

Surface skin is the most common site of this disease, and it is the easiest to cure. Other than superficial skin cancer, the most common sites are the lung, the breast, and the colon and rectum.

Because superficial skin cancer is so visible, it is usually found early. Left untreated, however, this kind of cancer can also cause death.

Stanley Robbins in *Pathology* describes various types of skin cancer:

1. *Basal cell cancer*—This is the most curable of all cancers. It has a 98 percent five-year survival rate.

2. *Epidermoid* or *squamous cell cancer*—This type is more serious than basal cell, because it has more of a tendency to spread to other parts of the body.[2]

Overexposure to the sun is the leading cause of skin cancer.

Malignant melanoma is not strictly "skin cancer," because it goes deeper than the skin and is more serious. It may have roots that penetrate deep into the body. It usually appears as a small, molelike growth that gets bigger.

Mycosis fungoides may involve other organs of the body. This is a form of lymphoma that affects the skin first. It appears as reddish, rounded tumors on the skin.[3]

CANCER OF THE LUNG

Lung cancer is the leading cause of cancer death in men. Scientists claim that this kind of cancer is largely preventable and that the primary cause of lung cancer is cigarette smoking.

Formerly lung cancer was rare in women, but for the first time more women are dying from lung cancer than breast cancer. In 1950, by contrast, lung cancer ranked seventh as a cause of cancer death in women. According to Robert McKenna, president of the American Cancer Society, the rise in lung cancer is due entirely to an increase in cigarette smoking among women.

Two-thirds of the people who undergo

surgery for lung cancer already have a metastatic tumor elsewhere in the body, so the survival rate is not as good as it could be if the disease were detected earlier.

CANCER OF THE BREAST

Breast cancer is a common type of cancer in women. It is seen occasionally in men and rarely in children.

Most lumps are discovered by self-examination, and most are not malignant. Early diagnosis is important, since it is vital to stop the growth of a malignancy before it spreads to another part of the body.

Surgery is the main treatment for breast cancer, sometimes in combination with chemotherapy and radiation therapy. The patient's ovaries may be removed, because some breast cancers are thought to be hormone-promoted.

Several different surgical procedures are used for breast cancer, and the most common ones are these:

1. *Extended radical mastectomy* or *supraradical mastectomy*—surgical removal of the entire breast, underlying chest muscles, the internal mammary chain of lymph nodes, and lymph nodes in the armpit.

2. *Modified radical mastectomy*—surgical removal of breast and lymph nodes in armpit.

3. *Simple* or *total mastectomy*—surgical removal of the breast, but none of the chest muscles or lymph nodes.

4. *Limited surgical procedures*—removal of the tumor mass and a varying amount of surrounding tissue. This type of procedure, sometimes called lumpectomy or tumorectomy, is controversial. It is generally reserved for extremely early breast cancer.

Most doctors recommend the radical or modified radical mastectomy, but many surgeons are now performing the initial surgery with techniques that will allow for reconstructive surgery later.

CANCER OF THE COLON AND RECTUM
The surgical treatment for this type of cancer is the removal of the bowel containing the tumor and adjoining tissue and the lymph nodes that drain the area. If extensive surgery of the rectum is necessary, a temporary or permanent opening in the abdominal wall can be used to eliminate waste. This is called a colostomy. After adjusting to the inconvenience of the colostomy bag, the patient can lead an otherwise normal, active life. Ask your doctor if there is an Ostomy Rehabilitation Program in your area.

The cause of this kind of cancer is unknown, but many scientists believe that the American diet—consisting of too much meat, not enough fiber, too much processing of foods—may have a great deal to do with it.

The following are some of the other common sites of cancer, listed alphabetically.

CANCER OF THE BONE

Bone cancer most often strikes children and young adults between the ages of ten and twenty. Relatively rare, it is usually diagnosed by biopsy, X-ray, and isotope scanning.

Bone cancer originates in the skeletal tissues. Very often the bone is a site of metastasis from another place in the body, usually breast, kidney, thyroid, or prostate.

CANCER OF THE BLADDER

Bladder cancer is the most frequent malignancy of the urinary tract. The two main types of cancer of the bladder are papillary and transitional-cell carcinoma. The papillary type is more common and is the more easily cured. If detected early, there is a good possibility of complete recovery.

CANCER OF THE BRAIN

Cancers of the brain vary widely in their rate of growth, as well as their physical and chemical processes. Survival depends greatly upon which type of tumor is involved.

Brain tumors are almost always treated by surgery, often followed by radiation. In the past, drugs have been less effective in treating cancer of the brain, because the protective membrane surrounding the brain could not be penetrated. New drugs have been developed, however, which are able to penetrate the "brain barrier." Researchers are also finding that using a combination of drugs can be effective.

Though seen most often in adults, brain cancer is the second most common cancer in children and has an especially high incidence in children aged five to nine.

CANCER OF THE LARYNX

Surviving cancer of the larynx, or voice box, depends almost entirely on how early it is discovered and treatment begun. The larynx is more accessible than some sites, and symptoms of this type of cancer (usually hoarseness) normally appear early, while the tumor is still small and localized. If the diagnosis is made early, when the cancer is limited to one vocal cord, the patient has a good chance of retaining the larynx.

Surgical removal of the larynx is necessary if the cancer has spread to other areas of the larynx and throat. Great strides have been made in rehabilitating laryngectomees, and across the country clubs have been formed by laryngectomees interested in helping others learn esophageal speech. This kind of speech is produced by expelling air from the esophagus, and the great majority of laryngectomees have found it so successful that they have been able to return to full employment and lead otherwise normal lives.

LEUKEMIA, LYMPHOMA, AND MULTIPLE MYELOMA

Leukemia is cancer of the blood-forming tissues. It originates in the bone marrow and it is not confined to a tumor in one place in the body.

The leukemia patient produces too many white cells. Normally the white blood cells help the body fight infection, but the leukemic cells are undifferentiated cells and do not possess this capability. These abnormal cells invade all the organs of the body.

Cancer takes the lives of more children under fifteen than any other disease, and over half of these are leukemia patients. The vast majority of children with leukemia have *acute lymphocytic* (or *lymphoblastic*) *leukemia*, and it is treated more successfully than other types, especially in younger school-age children.

The leukemia patient has new hope because of the promising research of this area. New drugs are available that help him stay in a state of remission where the bone marrow can function normally again, and he can be free of symptoms. Bone marrow transplants are also being done with some degree of success, though this is still an experimental procedure and there are many unanswered questions.

More than 90 percent of children with acute lymphocytic leukemia will go into remission. Then the patient is put on a program of drugs to keep him in remission. This is

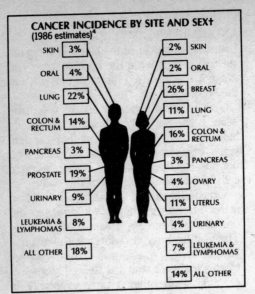

CANCER INCIDENCE BY SITE AND SEX†
(1986 estimates)[4]

SKIN	3%	2%	SKIN
ORAL	4%	2%	ORAL
LUNG	22%	26%	BREAST
COLON & RECTUM	14%	11%	LUNG
PANCREAS	3%	16%	COLON & RECTUM
PROSTATE	19%	3%	PANCREAS
URINARY	9%	4%	OVARY
LEUKEMIA & LYMPHOMAS	8%	11%	UTERUS
ALL OTHER	18%	4%	URINARY
		7%	LEUKEMIA & LYMPHOMAS
		14%	ALL OTHER

†Excluding non-melanoma skin cancer and carcinoma in situ.

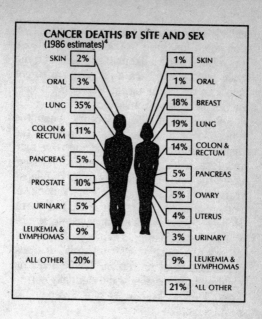

CANCER DEATHS BY SITE AND SEX
(1986 estimates)[4]

	Male		Female	
SKIN	2%	1%	SKIN
ORAL	3%	1%	ORAL
		18%	BREAST
LUNG	35%	19%	LUNG
COLON & RECTUM	11%	14%	COLON & RECTUM
PANCREAS	5%	5%	PANCREAS
PROSTATE	10%	5%	OVARY
URINARY	5%	4%	UTERUS
		3%	URINARY
LEUKEMIA & LYMPHOMAS	9%	9%	LEUKEMIA & LYMPHOMAS
ALL OTHER	20%	21%	ALL OTHER

called "maintenance therapy" and usually is continued for three to five years. If relapse (or return of the leukemia) should occur, the child will be put back on a program to get him into remission again. Each time it gets harder to achieve remission.

A state of remission occurs when the leukemia patient has no symptoms of the disease, and when the blood and bone marrow tests show no leukemia cells. Remission is not the same thing as being cured; relapse can always occur, since a certain number of leukemia cells, though unseen, are there. However, remissions are now lasting several years, and the patients can hope for the discovery of a permanent cure while in an extended state of remission. These leukemic children in remission lead essentially normal lives. They look good; they feel good; they go to school.

Chronic leukemia is an overproduction of all types of bone marrow cells, and it may be controlled for years.

Lymphatic leukemia may continue for twenty years or more.

The treatment for leukemia in general may include radiation therapy, radioactive phosphorus, and other drugs. Sometimes blood transfusions, platelet transfusions, and antibiotics are prescribed.

Hodgkin's disease and *lymphoma* are solid tumors of the lymph glands and are closely related to leukemia.

Multiple myeloma is a tumor of the bone,

which is characterized by a proliferation of plasma cells and may show bone and soft tissue tumors.

CANCER OF THE MOUTH
Oral cancer occurs most frequently on the lip, then on the cheek and tongue. Other common sites of cancer of the mouth are the floor of the mouth, gums, palate, tonsils, lower jaw, and salivary glands.

The most common symptom is a sore that does not heal. Surgery and radiation therapy are used for treatment of cancer of the mouth, and highly skilled techniques of reconstructive and plastic surgery can be used to help restore areas affected by radical surgery.

Mouth cancer is strongly associated with cigarette smoking, excessive drinking of alcohol in combination with cigarettes, chewing tobacco, and using snuff. It appears to be even more strongly linked with pipe and cigar smoking. Chronic irritation from such things as jagged teeth and poorly fitting dentures can also cause mouth cancer.

CANCER OF THE PROSTATE
Prostate cancer rarely strikes men under forty, but after age fifty-five it is the third leading cause of cancer death in men.

The prostate is a gland in the male genital

system. It is located just below the bladder. The symptoms for this kind of cancer usually involve urinary difficulty. If the growth is confined to the prostate alone, this gland is removed, and the chances for survival are excellent. If the symptoms become severe, and if there is evidence that the cancer is spreading, it is sometimes necessary to perform an orchiectomy (surgical removal of the testes) and administer hormone treatment.

CANCER OF THE STOMACH AND ESOPHAGUS

Stomach cancer is on the decline in this country, but the stomach is still a frequent site of the disease. Although scientists are not sure about the cause of stomach cancer, they tend to feel that diet is at least partially responsible.

Countries in which people consume great quantities of fish, such as Japan and Iceland, report a far higher stomach cancer incidence than the United States.

Esophageal cancer is fairly uncommon in the United States. It is usually treated by surgery, particularly if the tumor is in the lower portion of the esophagus. The portion of the esophagus removed by surgery can be reconstructed from a section of the colon. The upper portion of the esophagus can be treated by radiation. So far, anti-cancer drugs have not been found effective in treating esophageal cancer.

CANCER OF THE TESTES

Although testicular cancer accounts for only about 1 percent of all cancer in males, in men between the ages of twenty-nine and thirty-five it is the most common type of cancer. The prognosis after treatment for this type of cancer is excellent. The malignancy is nearly always confined to one testicle, and the remaining testicle usually retains complete fertility.

CANCER OF THE THYROID

Beginning in the 1920s and continuing for over twenty-five years, X rays were used to treat children and adolescents for such noncancerous conditions as ringworm, ear inflammations, inflammations of the sinuses, enlarged tonsils and adenoids, and acne. A link has been established between those X-ray treatments and an increased incidence in thyroid tumors in those people as adults.

Most of these thyroid tumors are benign, or noncancerous, and even when they are malignant, they are usually treated successfully.

CANCER OF THE UTERUS

The first visible signs of cancer of the uterus are irregular bleeding or unusual vaginal discharge. Irregularities in the menstrual cycle, profuse periods, and the recurrence of a period after several months without periods are additional symptoms.

Uterine cancer may be treated by radiation therapy or surgery, or a combination of the two. Drugs, such as synthetic hormones, are also used in treating advanced cancer of the uterus. Surgery is performed to remove all of the cancerous tissue or the organ itself. If complete removal of the growth is not possible, surgery may still help to make the patient more comfortable and extend her life.

To obtain more detailed information about the type of cancer you are facing, contact your nearest branch of the American Cancer Society. You will probably find the telephone listing under the name of your county in the white pages of your directory.

Helping Agencies

1. *American Cancer Society Helpline* (1-800-ACS-2345) operates from 9:00 A.M. to 5:00 P.M. After-hour calls are recorded. Available in states east of and including Kansas.

2. *Cancer Information Service* (1-800-4-CANCER) operates from 9:00 A.M. to 5:00 P.M. and is funded by the National Cancer Institute. In Alaska, dial 1-800-638-6070; in Hawaii, call collect 808-524-1234; and in Washington, D.C., call 202-635-5700.

3. *Reach to Recovery* provides support for women who have had breast surgery or are now facing it. Call your local American Cancer Society office for information, or write Reach to Recovery, American Cancer Society, Inc., 777 Third Ave., New York, New York 10017.

NOTES

CHAPTER 1
1. *Everything You Always Wanted to Know about Cancer but Were Afraid to Ask* (n.p.: United Cancer Council, n.d.), p. 3.
2. *Answering Your Questions about Cancer* (New York: American Cancer Society, 1971), p. 6.

CHAPTER 2
1. Pat McGrady, *Science against Cancer* (New York: Public Affairs Pamphlets, 1962), p. 13.
2. Susan Golden, "Cancer Chemotherapy and Management of Patient Problems," *Nursing Forum 14* no. 3 (1975): 279-280.

CHAPTER 3
1. James Dobson, *Hide or Seek* (Old Tappan, N.J.: Revell, 1974), p. 15.
2. Rene C. Mastrovito, "Cancer: Awareness and Denial," Memorial Sloan-Kettering Cancer Center *Clinical Bulletin 4*, no. 4 (1974): 142.
3. Eileen Tiedt, "The Psychodynamic Process of the Oncological Experience," *Nursing Forum 14*, no. 3 (1975): 268.
4. Mastrovito, p. 142.
5. Maurice E. Wagner, *The Sensation of Being Somebody* (Grand Rapids: Zondervan, 1975), p. 146.

6. Mastrovito, p. 142.

7. Mastrovito, p. 143.

8. Dobson, p. 135.

CHAPTER 4

1. Darien B. Cooper, *You Can Be the Wife of a Happy Husband* (Wheaton, Ill.: Victor, 1974), p. 108.

2. Eileen Tiedt, "The Psychodynamic Process of the Oncological Experience," *Nursing Forum 14*, no. 3 (1975): 268.

3. Cooper, p. 106.

4. "Coping with Life's Strains," *U.S. News and World Report*, 1 May 1978, p. 82.

5. Tim LaHaye, *How to Win Over Depression* (Grand Rapids: Zondervan, 1974), pp. 53-54.

CHAPTER 5

1. Cicely Saunders, *The Management of Terminal Illness* (n.p.: Hospital Medicine Publications, n.d.), p. 23.

2. Ibid., p. 24.

3. Cicely Saunders, "Control of Pain in Terminal Cancer," *Nursing Times, Care of the Dying* 2d ed., 1976, p. 13.

4. Ibid.

5. Joseph Bayly, *The View from a Hearse* (Elgin, Ill.: Cook, 1969), p. 88.

APPENDIX

1. Most of the information in this section is from the publications of the Public Health Service, National Institutes of Health, United States Department of Health, Education, and Welfare, Washington, D.C. 20402.

2. Stanley Robbins, *Pathology* 3d ed. (Philadelphia: Saunders, 1967), pp. 1298, 1301, 1309.

3. Ibid., p. 1353.

4. "1986 Cancer Facts and Figures" (New York: American Cancer Society, 1986), p. 12.

About the Author

MARY BETH MOSTER is a free-lance writer and part-time lecturer at the Indiana University School of Journalism. She is the author of *When Mom Goes to Work* (Moody) and coauthor of *The Valley Is Bright* (Nelson). She, her husband, Stephen, and their three children live in central Indiana.